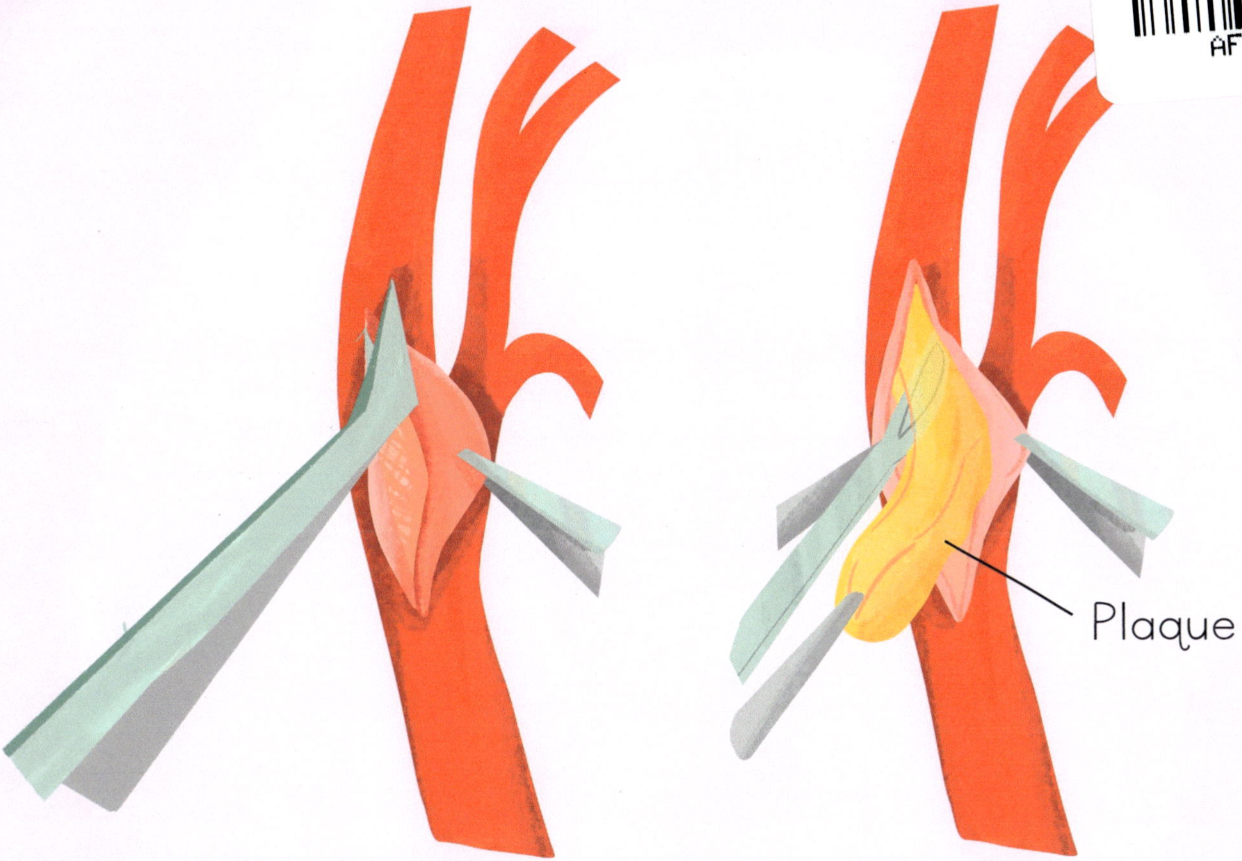

Artery opened

Plaque removed

Atherosclerosis can also be treated by scraping plaques off the wall of arteries. This is called **endarterectomy**.

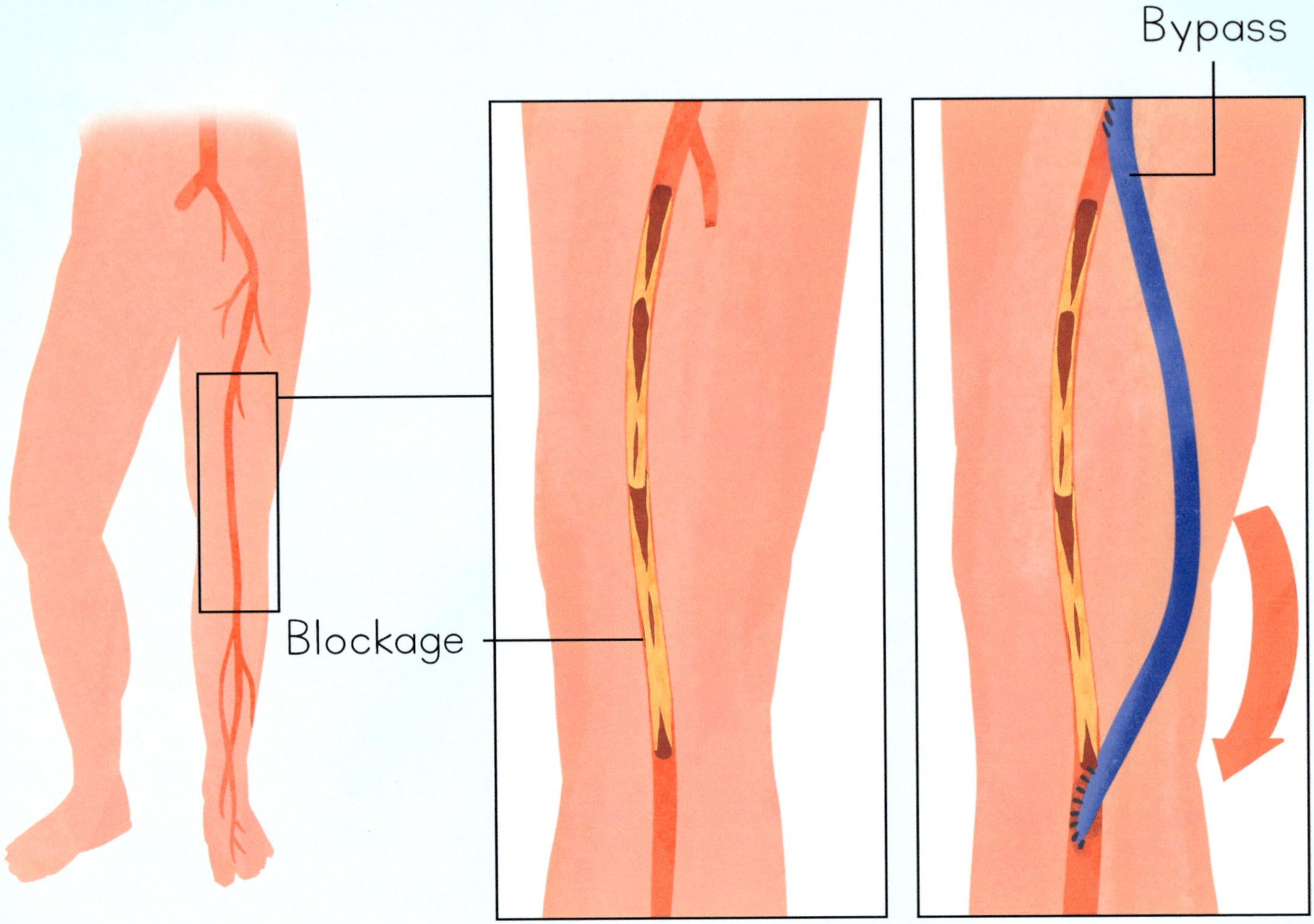

Some areas of blockage are so large that the best way to improve blood flow is to create a completely new route for the blood. This is called a **bypass**.

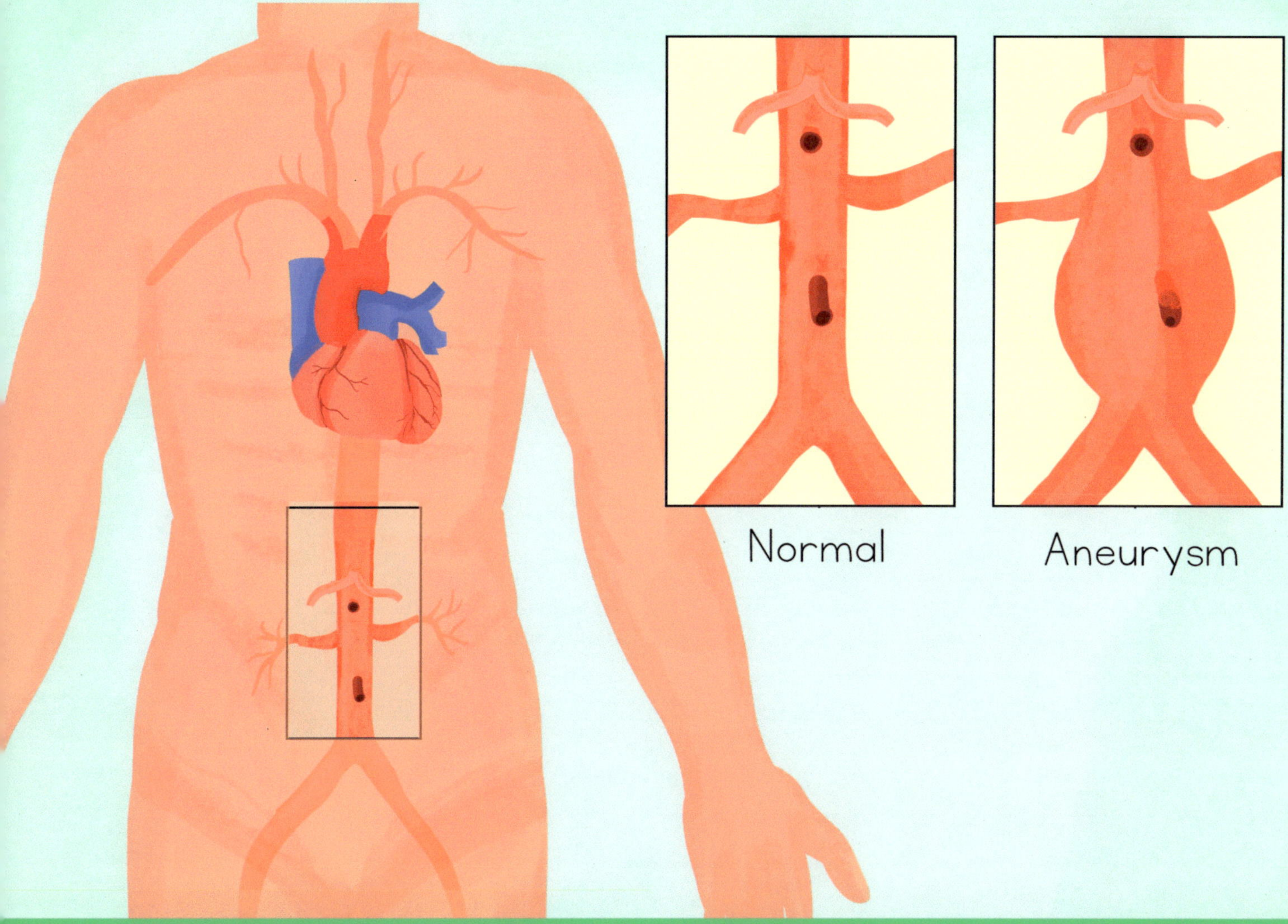

Sometimes, artery walls become weak and stretch out like a balloon, causing an **aneurysm**. The larger an aneurysm gets, the more likely it is to burst.

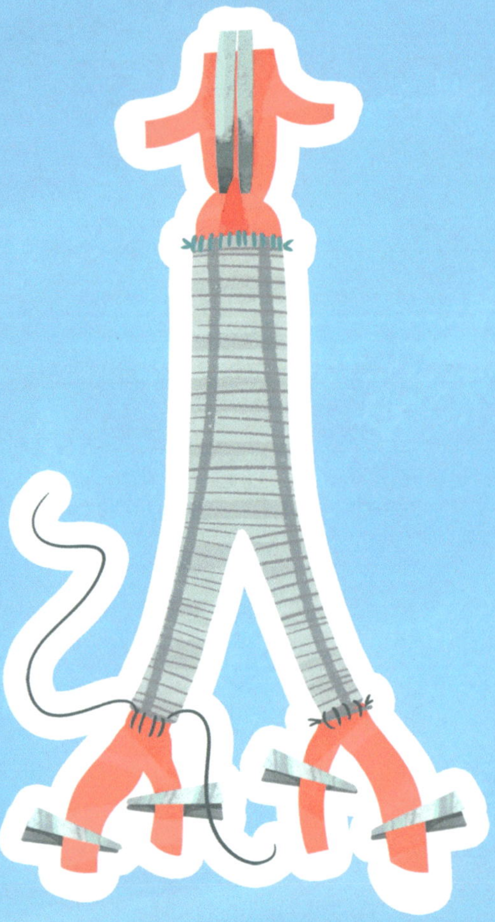

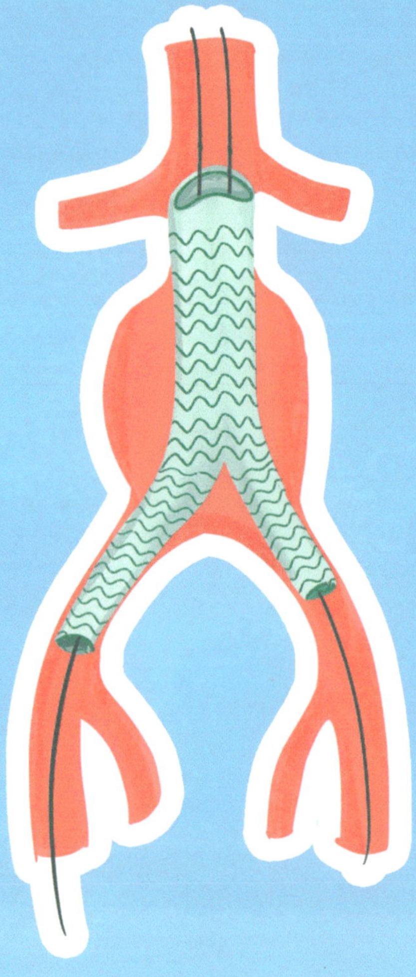

Aneurysms can be repaired with grafts that are sewn to replace the artery or with stents that have a fabric covering to reline the artery.

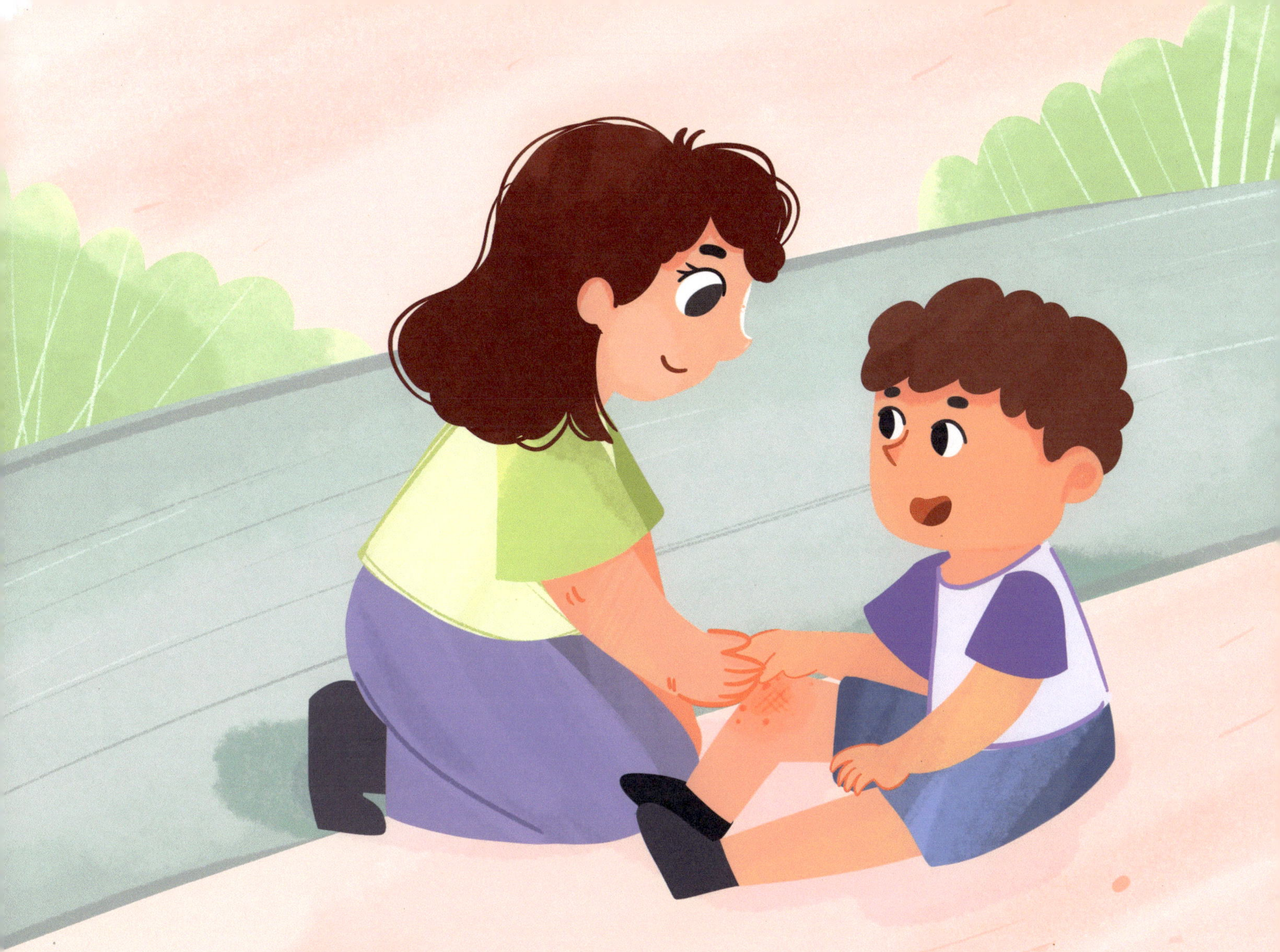

Sometimes, blood can stick to itself, forming **clots**. If we scrape our knee, clots stop the bleeding, but clots can also form when we don't want them.

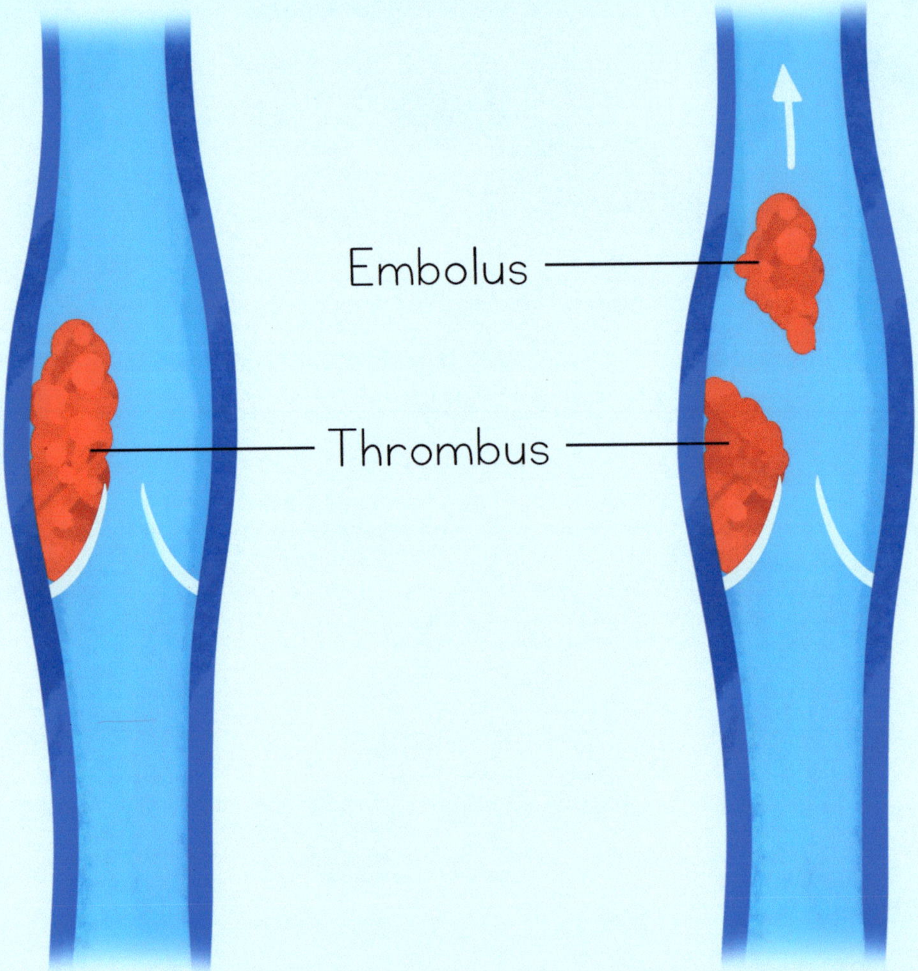

A **thrombus** is a blood clot that forms in a blood vessel and stays there. An **embolus** is a blood clot that breaks off and travels somewhere else.

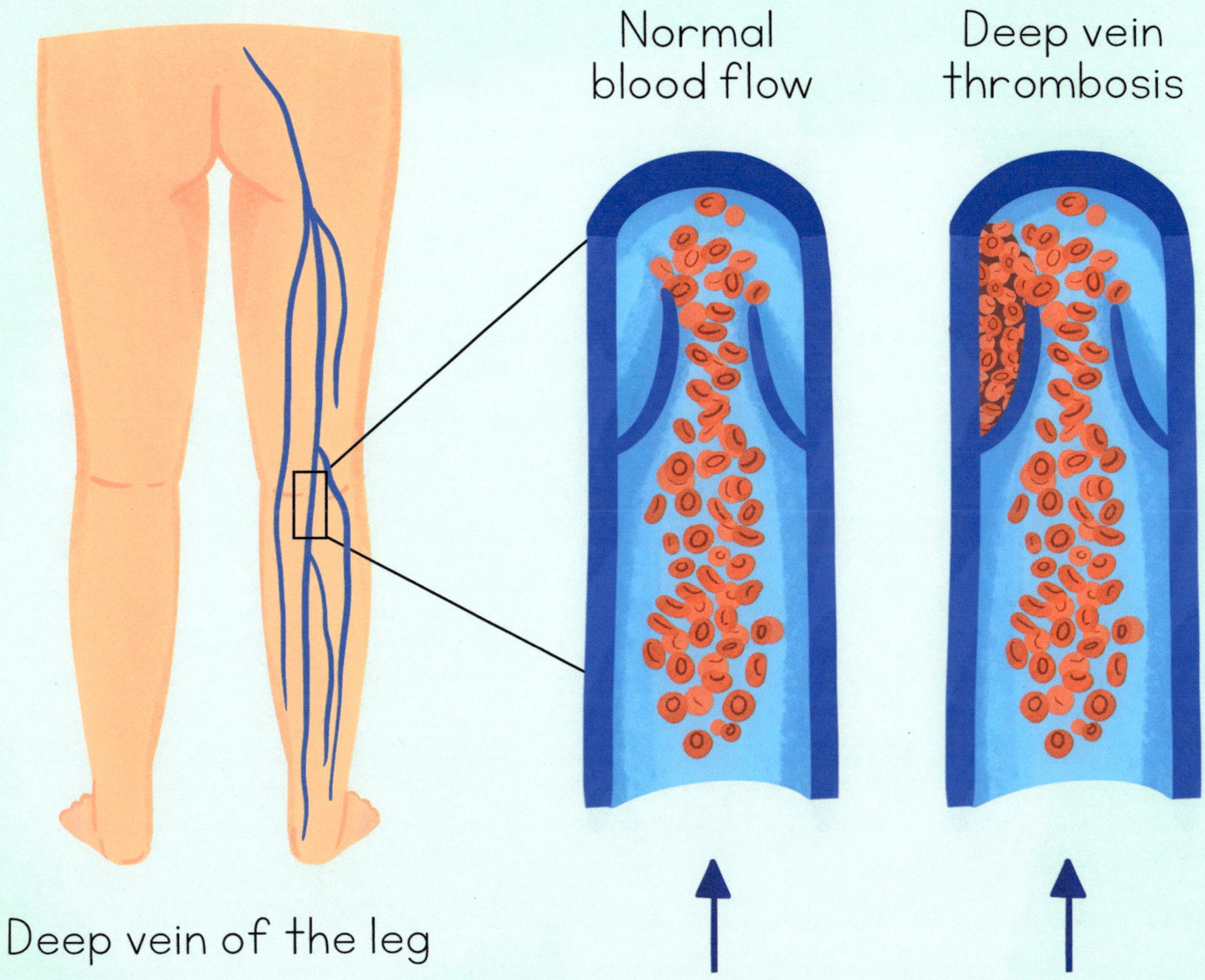

People can develop clots in the deep leg veins, especially if they do not walk or move around for many hours. This is called a **deep vein thrombosis**.

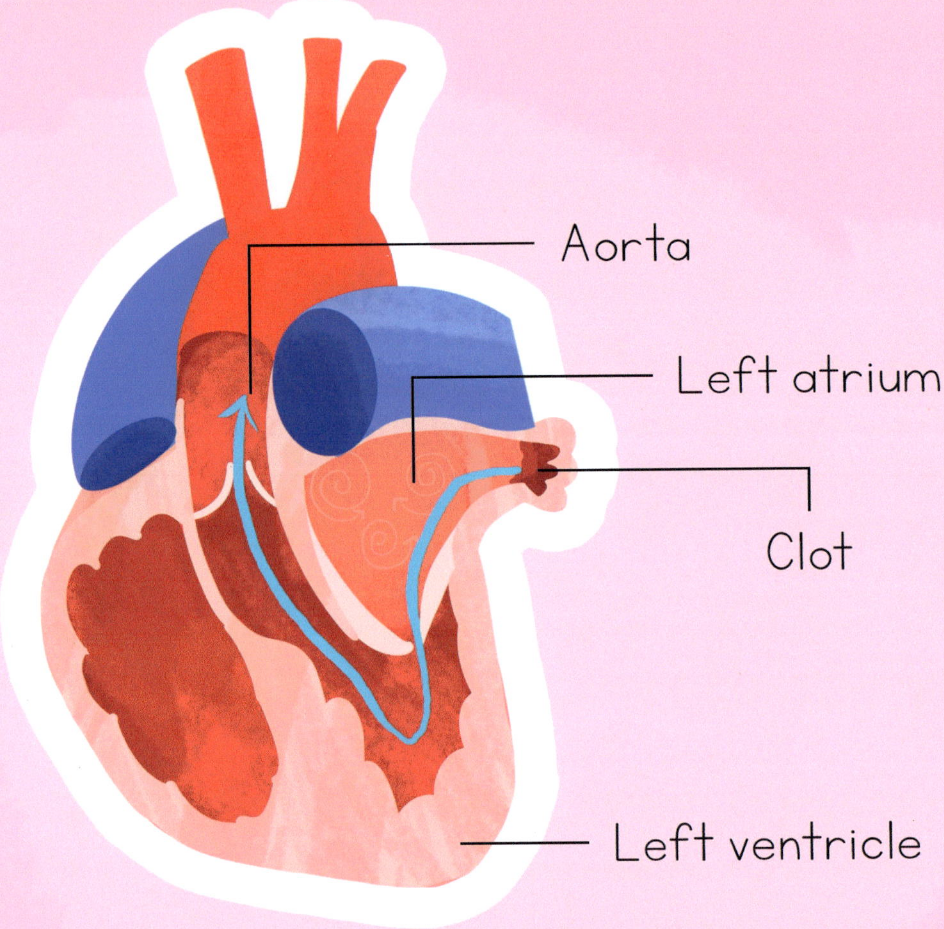

Some people have a type of irregular heart beat, called **atrial fibrillation**, that can cause blood clots to form in the heart and travel to the arteries.

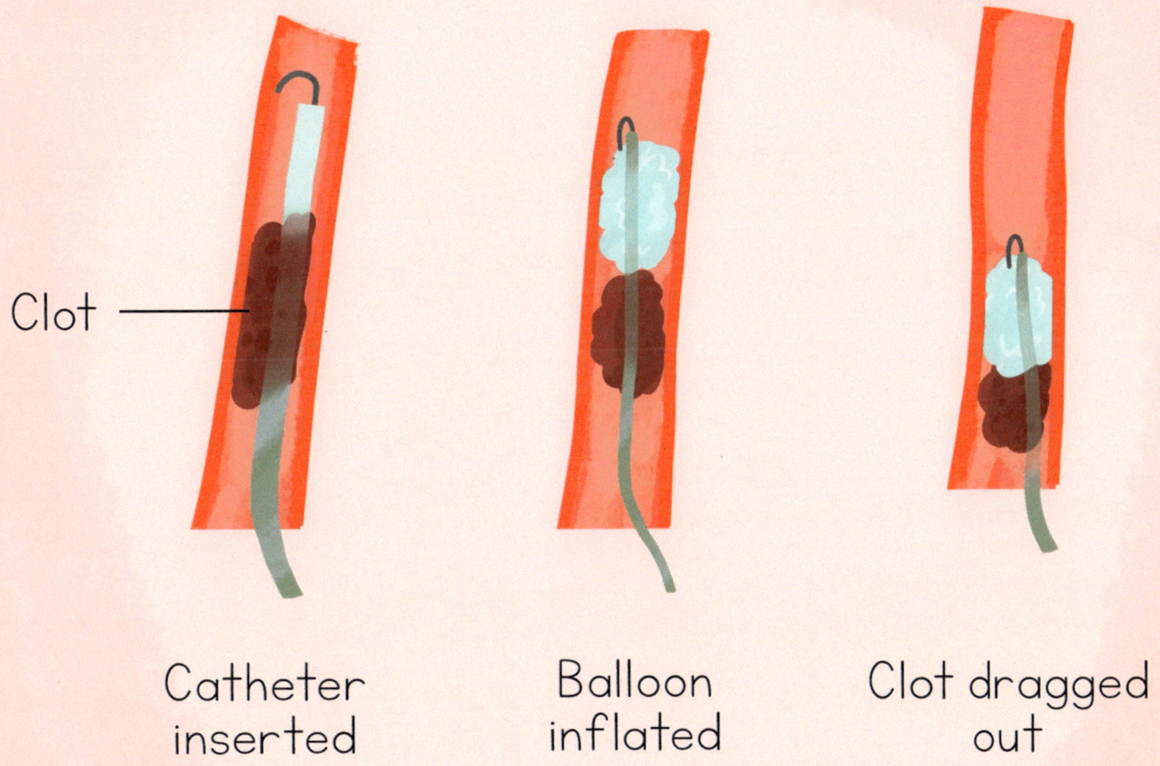

Blood clots can be removed by inflating a balloon to drag them out. This is called **thrombectomy**.

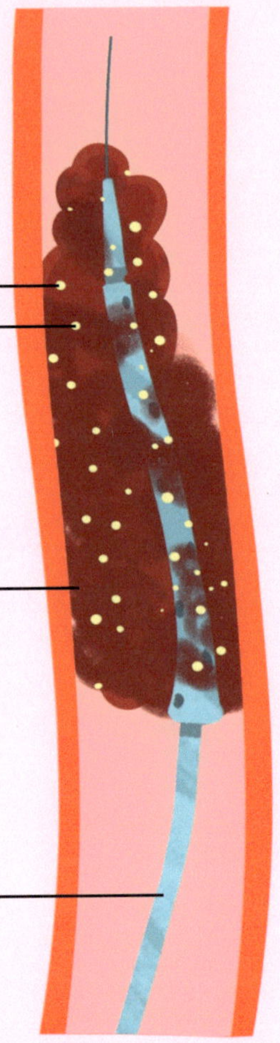

Bloods clots can also be dissolved using special medications delivered through a catheter. This is called **thrombolysis**.

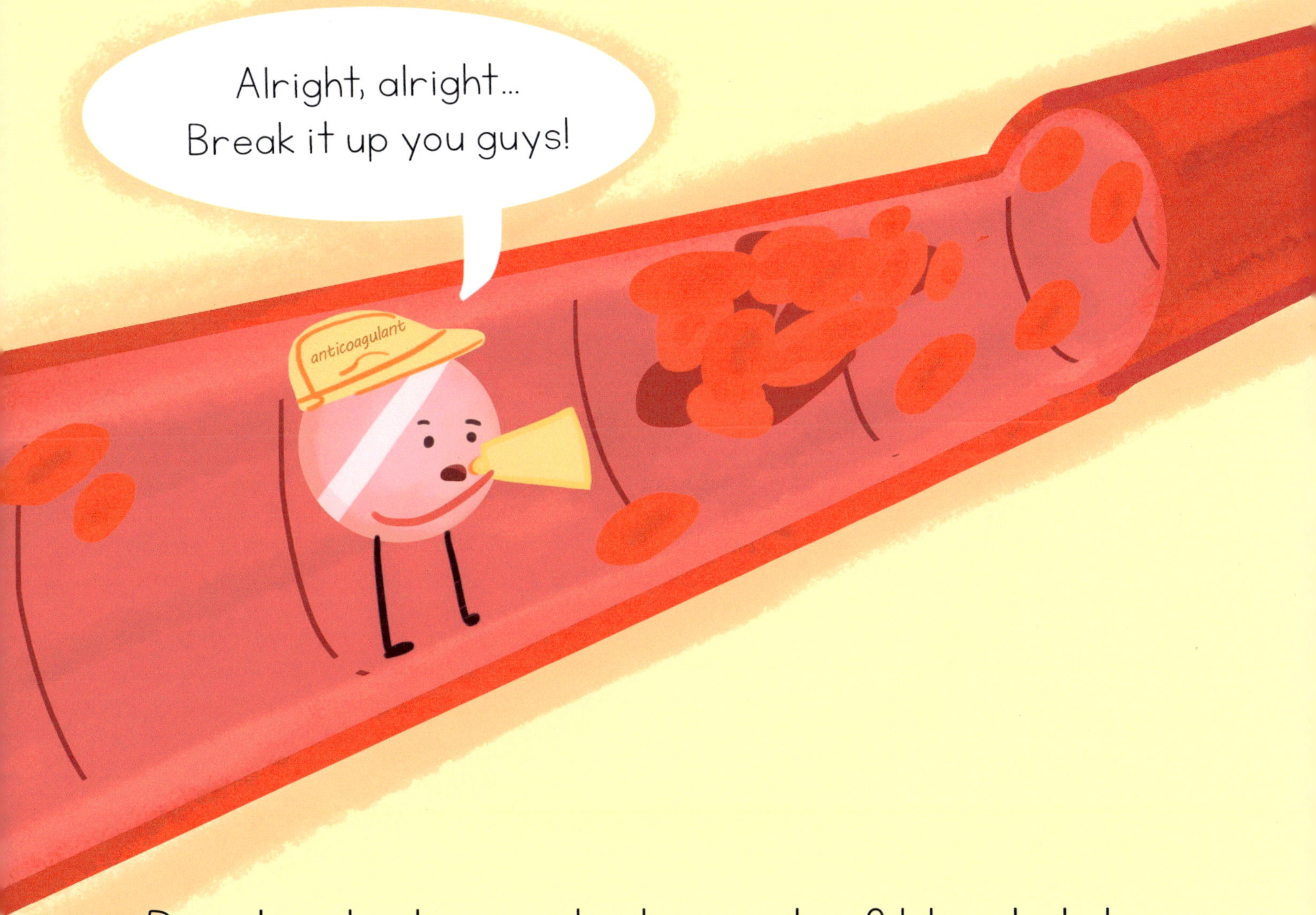

People who have a higher risk of blood clots can take medications called **anticoagulants** to help keep their blood flowing smoothly.

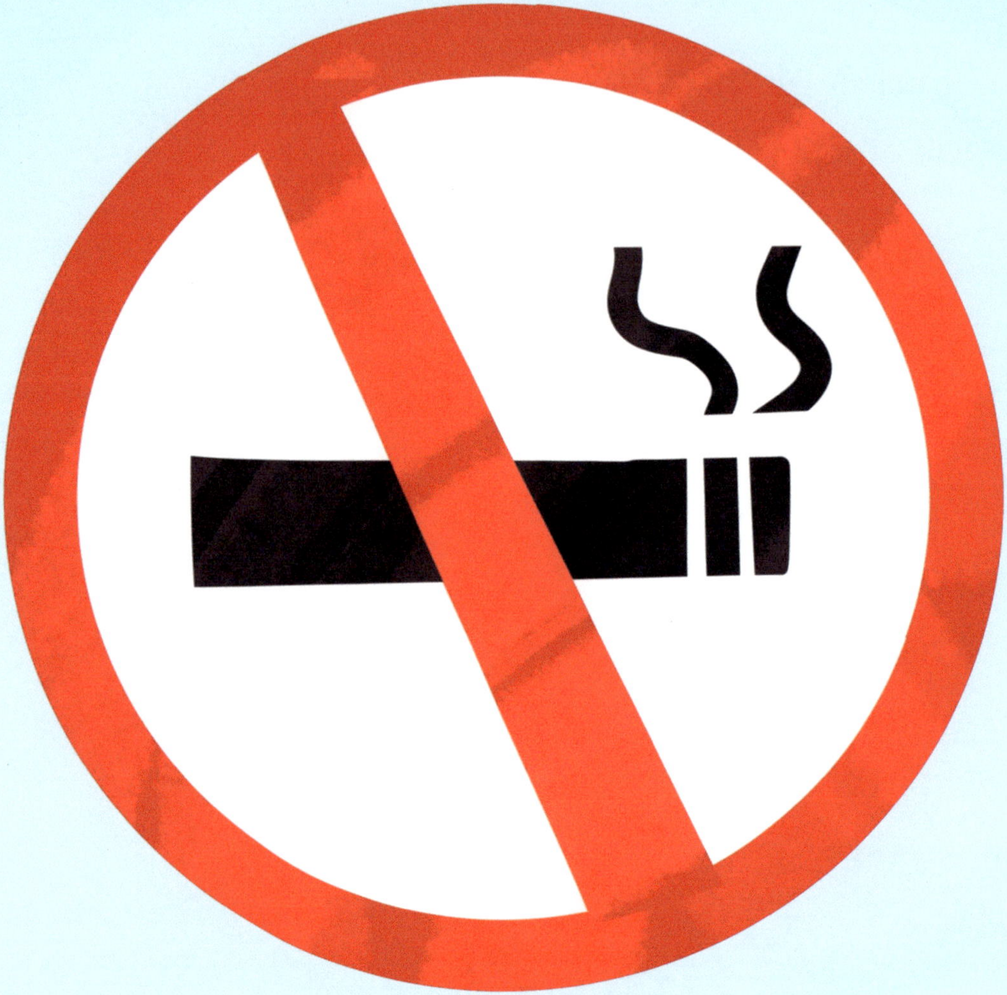

Smoking severely damages blood vessels. Over time, smoking can cause serious problems such as atherosclerosis, aneurysms, and clots.

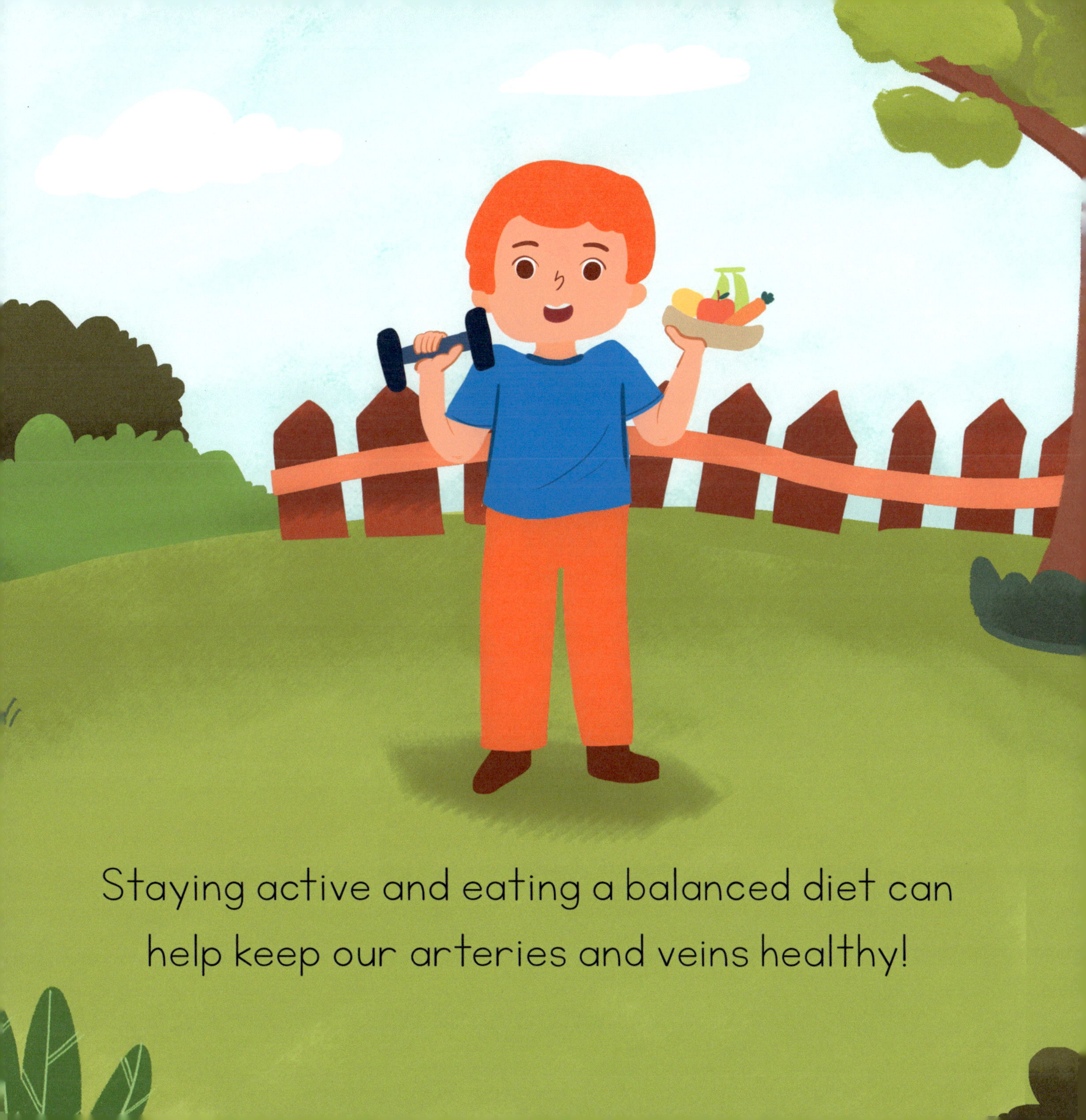

Staying active and eating a balanced diet can help keep our arteries and veins healthy!

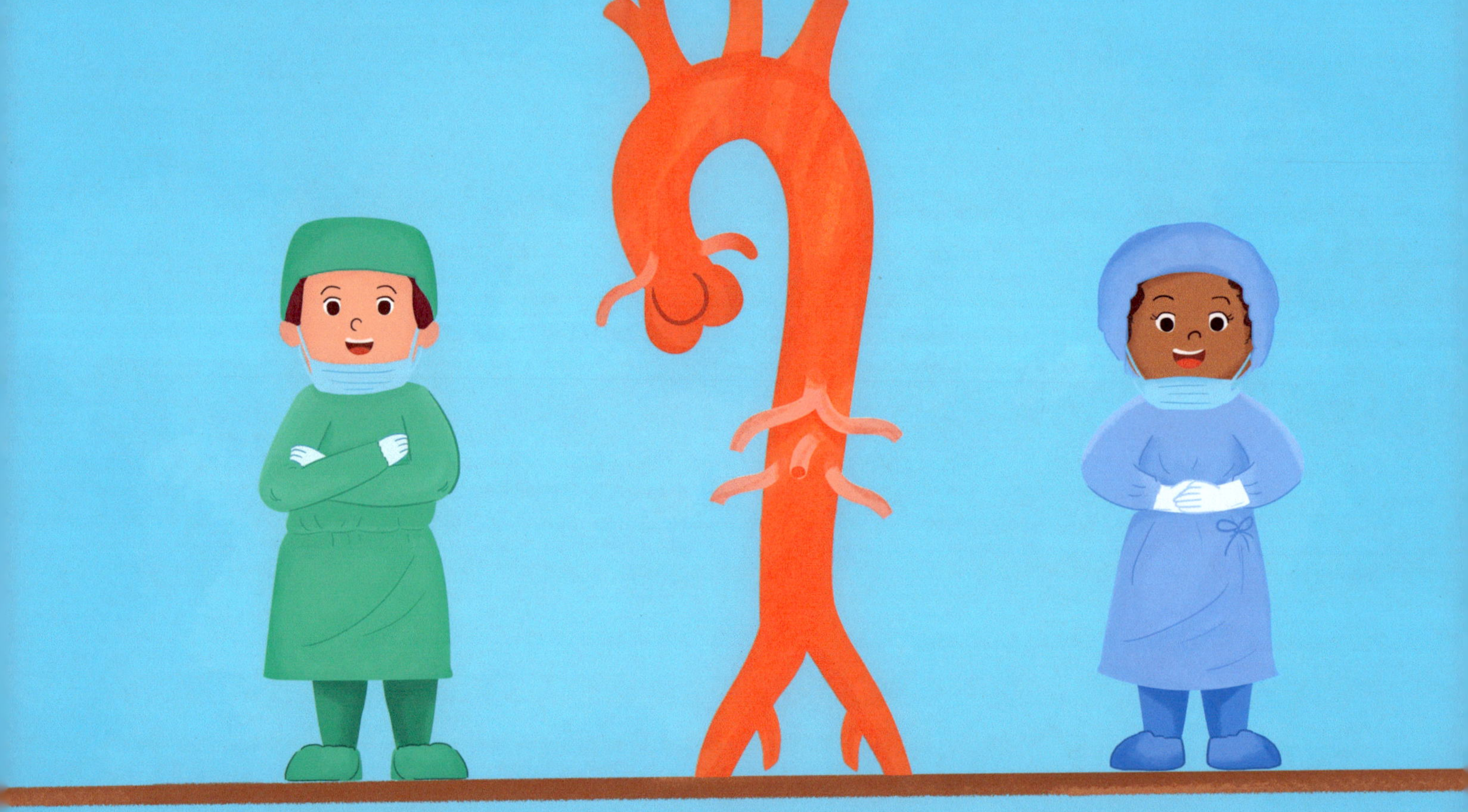

YOU'RE A FUTURE VASCULAR SURGEON!

Glossary

Aneurysm (A-nyr-i-zm): weakened artery or vein wall that stretches out
Angiogram (AN-jee-uh-gram): picture of blood vessels made by injecting contrast and taking x-rays
Anticoagulants (an-tee-kow-A-gyuh-luhnts): medications that prevent clots
Arteries (AAR-tr-eez): elastic tubes that carry blood away from the heart
Atherosclerosis (a-thr-ow-sklr-OW-suhs): plaque in arteries that causes **ischemia**, or reduced blood flow; can affect arteries that supply the **heart** (**coronary artery disease**, which can cause **angina**), the limbs (**peripheral artery disease**), and the brain (**carotid artery disease**, which can cause **stroke**); treated with medications (**statins**) or procedures (e.g. **angioplasty** and **stenting, endarterectomy**, **bypass**)
Atrial fibrillation (AY-tree-uhl fi-bruh-LAY-shn): irregular heart beat that can lead to formation of blood clots in the heart that travel in arteries
Clot (klaat): lump of blood that stops bleeding; can form in a blood vessel and stay there (**thrombus**) or travel to another part of the body (**embolus**); can be removed by inflating a balloon to drag it out (**thrombectomy**) or by delivering medications to dissolve it (**thrombolysis**)
Deep vein thrombosis (thraam-BOW-suhs): clot that forms in deep veins
Pulse (puhls): expansion of an artery that you can feel in your body
Ultrasound (UHL-truh-sownd): sound waves used to make pictures of structures inside the body, including blood vessels
Veins (vaynz): thin-walled tubes that carry blood *toward* the heart

Let's review what you learned!

1. What type of blood vessel carries blood away from the heart?
2. What type of blood vessel carries blood toward the heart?
3. What are two ways doctors can visualize blood vessels in our body?
4. What is plaque that can build up in the inner wall of arteries called?
5. What is reduced blood flow to a part of the body called?
6. What is atherosclerosis in arteries that supply the heart called?
7. What is chest pain or discomfort caused by coronary artery disease called?
8. What is atherosclerosis in arteries that supply the limbs called?
9. What is atherosclerosis in the carotid arteries called? What problem in the brain can this cause?
10. What medications can reduce the risk of developing problems from atherosclerosis? What three procedures can treat atherosclerosis?
11. What is a ballooning and weakened area in an artery called? What are two ways this can be repaired?
12. What is a blood clot that forms in a blood vessel and stays there called?
13. What is a blood clot that breaks off and travels somewhere else called?
14. What condition can cause blood clots to form in the heart?
15. What are blood clots in deep veins of the leg called?
16. What medications can reduce the risk of developing blood clots? What are two ways blood clots can be treated?
17. What are three ways we can keep our arteries and veins healthy?

Your Answers

1. ______________________________
2. ______________________________
3. ______________________________
4. ______________________________
5. ______________________________
6. ______________________________
7. ______________________________
8. ______________________________
9. ______________________________
10. ______________________________
11. ______________________________
12. ______________________________
13. ______________________________
14. ______________________________
15. ______________________________
16. ______________________________
17. ______________________________

Answer Key

1. Arteries
2. Veins
3. Ultrasound and angiograms
4. Atherosclerosis
5. Ischemia
6. Coronary artery disease
7. Angina
8. Peripheral artery disease
9. Carotid artery disease; stroke
10. Statins; angioplasty and stenting, endarterectomy, and bypass
11. Aneurysm; sewn graft or stent graft
12. Thrombus
13. Embolus
14. Atrial fibrillation
15. Deep vein thrombosis
16. Anticoagulants; thrombectomy or thrombolysis
17. Don't smoke, stay active, and eat a balanced diet

Medical School FOR KIDS™

About the Authors

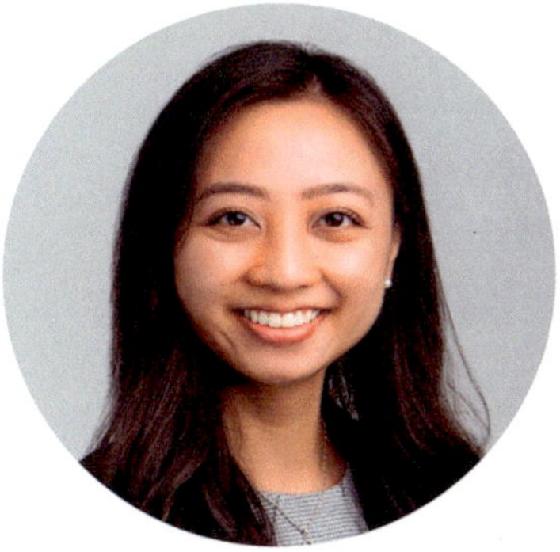

Betty Nguyen

Betty is a physician specializing in dermatology. She was born in Southern California but spent much of her childhood in Georgia, where she grew up on a chicken farm. Betty studied Biology at UCLA, where she was a Gates Millennium Scholar, and earned her MD from UC Riverside on a full-tuition scholarship. Outside of work, Betty is a certified yoga instructor and licensed scuba diver. She also enjoys journalistic writing and cycling.

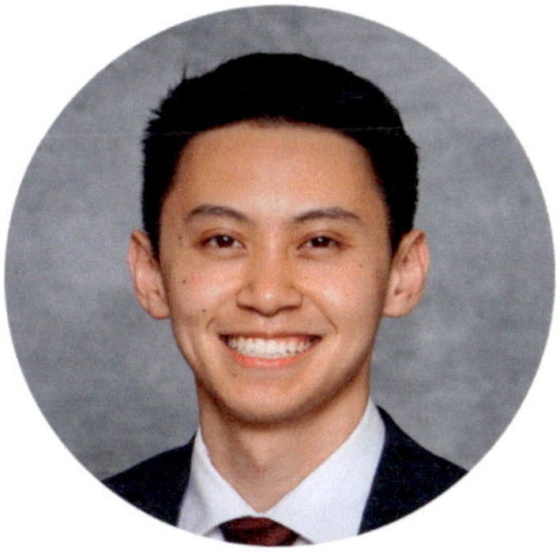

Brandon Pham

Brandon is a physician specializing in ophthalmology. He was born and raised in Southern California. Brandon studied Microbiology, Immunology, and Molecular Genetics at UCLA, where he was a Barry Goldwater Scholar, and earned his MD from Stanford. He is passionate about medical education for students of all ages. In his free time, Brandon enjoys traveling, playing tennis, and performing card magic tricks.

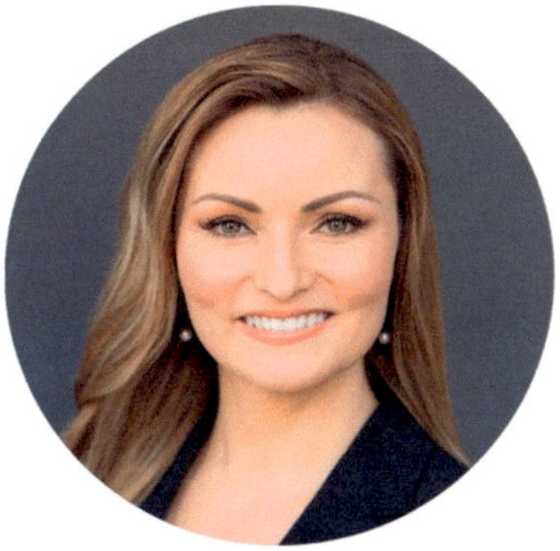

Samantha Stradleigh

Samantha is a physician specializing in vascular surgery. She was born and raised in Berkeley, California. She studied Chemical and Biomolecular Engineering at Cornell University and worked in Florida developing drug-eluting coronary stents. Samantha received her MD from Albert Einstein College of Medicine and then returned to California to complete her residency in vascular surgery at UC Davis. She has two young boys and enjoys teaching them about engineering and medicine.

Check out the rest of the books in our series!

Website: mdforkids.org

Instagram: @md.for.kids

Medical School FOR KIDS™

Made in the USA
Las Vegas, NV
10 November 2026

57843571R00026